'Mudras for Anxiety'

25 Simple Hand Gestures for Curing Anxiety

Advait

Disclaimer and FTC Notice

Mudras for Anxiety: 25 Simple Hand Gestures for Curing Anxiety
Copyright © 2014, Advait. All Rights Reserved.

ISBN-13: 978-1512242317

ISBN-10: 1512242314

The intent of the author is only to offer information of a general nature to help you in your quest for emotional, spiritual and physical well being. In the event you use any of the information in this book for yourself, which is your constitutional right, the author and the publisher assume no responsibility for your actions.

Under no circumstances will any legal responsibility or blame be held against the publisher for any reparation, damages, or monetary loss due to the information herein, either directly or indirectly. The information herein is offered for informational purposes solely, and is universal as so. The presentation of the information is without contract or any type of guarantee assurance.

Adherence to all applicable laws and regulations, including international, federal, state, and local governing professional licensing, business practices, advertising, and all other aspects of doing business in the US, Canada, or any other jurisdiction is the sole responsibility of the purchaser or reader.

Neither the author nor the publisher assumes any responsibility or liability whatsoever on the behalf of the purchaser or reader of these materials.

Any perceived slight of any individual or organization is purely unintentional.

Advait

Contents

Mudras for Anxiety

What are Mudras?

According to the Vedic culture of ancient India, our entire world is made of 'the five elements' called as *The Panch-Maha-Bhuta's*. The five elements being **Earth**, **Water**, **Fire**, **Wind** and **Space/Vacuum**. They are also called the earth element, water element, fire element, wind element and space element.

These five elements constitute the human body – the nutrients from the soil (earth) are absorbed by the plants which we consume (thus we survive on the earth element), the blood flowing through own veins represents the water element, the body heat represents the fire element, the oxygen we inhale and the carbon dioxide we exhale represents the wind element and the sinuses we have in our nose and skull represent the space element.

As long as these five elements in our body are balanced and maintain appropriate levels we remain healthy. An imbalance of these elements in the human body leads to a deteriorated health and diseases.

Now understand this, the command and control center of all these five elements lies in our fingers. So literally, our health lies at our fingertips.

The Mudra healing method that I am going to teach you depends on our fingers.

To understand this, we should first know the finger-element relationship:

Thumb – Fire element.

Index finger – Wind element.

Middle finger – Space/Vacuum element.

Third finger – Earth element.

Small finger – Water element.

This image will give you a better understanding of the concept:

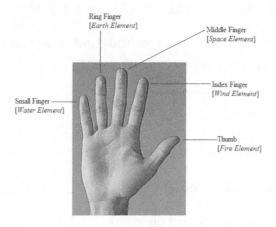

Ring Finger
[*Earth Element*]

Middle Finger
[*Space Element*]

Index Finger
[*Wind Element*]

Small Finger
[*Water Element*]

Thumb
[*Fire Element*]

When the fingers are brought together in a specific pattern and are touched to each other, or slightly pressed against each other, the formation is called as a *'Mudra'*.

When the five fingers are touched and pressed in a peculiar way to form a Mudra, it affects the levels of the five elements in our body, thus balancing those elements and inducing good health.

P.S. The Mudra Healing Methods aren't just theory or wordplay; these are healing methods from the ancient Indian Vedic culture, proven and tested over ages.

Attention!!

Read this before you read any further

For the better understanding of the reader, detail images have been provided for every mudra along with the method to perform it.

Most of the Mudras given in this book are to be performed using both your hands, but the Mudras whose images show only one hand performing the Mudra, are to be performed simultaneously on both your hands for the Mudras to have the maximum effect.

How to Use these Mudras?

The Mudras Mentioned in this book for curing anxiety can be classified into two categories, viz.

   a) Primary Mudras for curing Anxiety and,
   b) Secondary Mudras for Emotional Support, Stability & Confidence.

The Primary Mudras are the first 15 Mudras while the remaining 10 Mudras are the secondary Mudras.

The Primary Mudras are to be used directly and extensively for curing your Anxiety and the Secondary Mudras are to be used for garnering the required emotional support and stability during the course of Self-Healing and these secondary Mudras increase the healing effects of the Primary Mudras manifolds.

Make sure that you perform all the Primary Mudras regularly and extensively, while performing a few Secondary Mudras regularly which will enhance the effect of the Primary Mudras.

Also, understand that it is NOT a hard and fast rule that you should perform all these 25 Mudras back to back in one session.

Advait

Take your time, and perform these Mudras at your own pace and convenience.

The beauty of Mudra Health and Healing Techniques is that Mudras can be performed at any time and place: while stuck in traffic, at the office, watching TV, or whenever you have to twiddle your thumbs waiting for something or someone.

So, please don't come up with any excuses to avoid them, Mudras are as Easy and Effortless as Curing Anxiety can get.

Mudra #1

Dnyaanmudra / Mudra of Wisdom

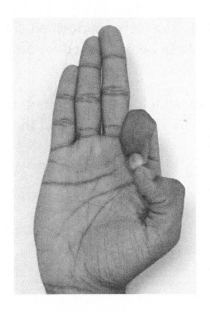

Method:

This Mudra is to be performed in a seated position.

Be seated comfortably in an upright posture and concentrate on your breathing to relax.

Join the tips of your Index finger and Thumb together and press slightly.

Advait

Keep all the other fingers extended outwards as shown in the image.

After forming the Mudras on both the hands, rest the Mudras on your thighs, palms facing up.

Duration:

This Mudra should be performed for at least 5 minutes and can be performed for 20 minutes at a stretch.

This Mudra should be performed twice a day, once in the morning and once in the evening for best results.

Mudra #2

Mushtimudra / Mudra of Fist

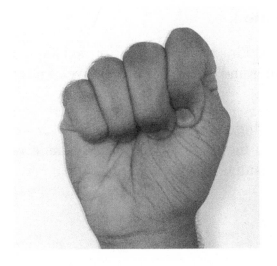

Method:

This Mudra is to be performed in a seated position.

Be seated comfortably in an upright posture and concentrate on your breathing to relax.

Touch the tip of your thumb to the base of the Ring finger and press slightly.

Advait

Close all the other fingers over the Thumb to form a fist.

(Refer the image)

Form this Mudra on each hand and rest the fists against the lower belly.

Duration:

This Mudra should be performed for at least 5 minutes and can be performed for 40 minutes at a stretch.

This Mudra should be performed twice a day, once in the morning and once in the evening for best results.

Mudra #3

Panchamukhmudra / Mudra of Five Faces

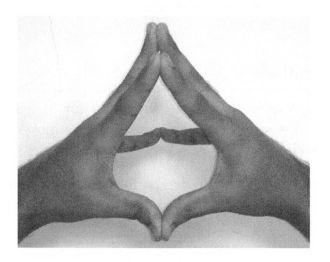

Method:

This Mudra is to be performed in a seated position.

Be seated comfortably in an upright posture and concentrate on your breathing to relax.

Hold your palms in front of your chest facing each other.

Advait

Now extend all the fingers on both the hands outwards.

Then, touch tips of all fingers of one hand to the tips of the respective fingers of the other hand. (refer the image)

Press the tips slightly.

Once the Mudra is formed lower the Mudra hold it in front of your abdomen.

Duration:

This Mudra should be performed for at least 5 minutes and can be performed for 20 minutes at a stretch.

This Mudra should be performed twice a day, once in the morning and once in the evening for best results.

Mudra #4

Rudramudra / Mudra of Lord Shiva

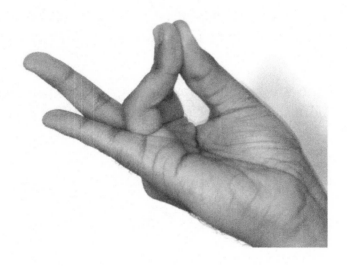

Method:

This Mudra is to be performed in a seated position.

Be seated comfortably in an upright posture and concentrate on your breathing to relax.

Place your hands on your thighs with your palms facing upwards.

Advait

Touch the tip of your Thumb with the tip of your Index finger and the tip of the Ring finger, press slightly.

Refer the image for more clarity.

Duration:

This Mudra should be performed for at least 5 minutes and can be performed for 40 minutes at a stretch.

If you are serious about losing weight then this Mudra should be performed at least 4 times a day.

Mudra #5

Shaktimudra / Mudra of Divine Feminine

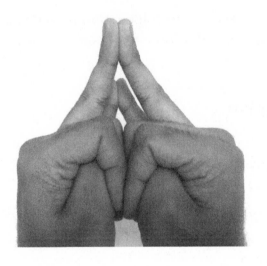

Method:

This Mudra is to be performed in a seated position.

Be seated comfortably in an upright posture and concentrate on your breathing to relax.

Advait

Keep your palms facing each other in front of your chest.

Then touch the tips of both your Little fingers and press slightly.

After that, touch the tips of both your Ring fingers and press slightly.

Fold your thumbs in to your palms

And, cover up the folded thumbs curling down your Index and Middle fingers into your palms.

Duration:

This Mudra should be performed for at least 5 minutes and can be performed for 40 minutes at a stretch.

This Mudra should be performed twice a day, once in the morning and once in the evening for best results.

Mudra #6

Shukrimudra / Mudra of Purity

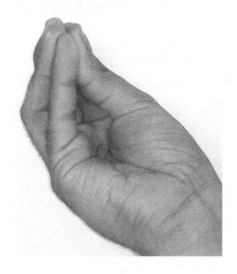

Method:

This Mudra can be performed while being seated, in a standing position or lying in bed.

Concentrate on your breathing to relax and feel comfortable.

Join the tips of all your fingers together to make this Mudra. (Refer the image)

Advait

Your palms should be facing upwards.

For best results perform this Mudra lying down.

Duration:

This Mudra should be performed for at least 5 minutes and can be performed for 30 minutes at a stretch.

This Mudra should be performed twice a day, once in the morning and once in the evening for best results.

Mudra #7

Dwitiiya Abhaymudra / Mudra of Assurance II

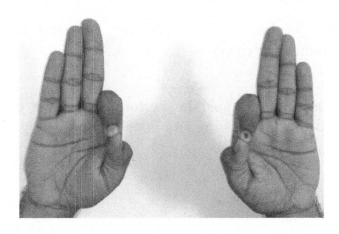

Method:

This Mudra is to be performed in a seated position.

Be seated comfortably in an upright posture and concentrate on your breathing to relax.

Bring your palms at shoulder height; make them face forward (away from your face).

Advait

Join the tips of the Thumb and Index finger on both hands, and press slightly.

Keep all the other fingers extended upwards.

Hold this Mudra at shoulder height at the same time relaxing your shoulders.

Duration:

This Mudra should be performed for at least 5 minutes and can be performed for 40 minutes at a stretch.

This Mudra should be performed twice a day, once in the morning and once in the evening for best results.

Mudra #8

PurnaDnyaanmudra / Mudra of Complete Wisdom

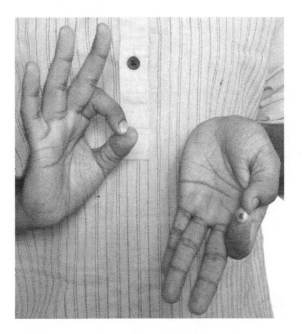

Method:

This Mudra is to be performed in a seated position.

Be seated comfortably in an upright posture and concentrate on your breathing to relax.

Advait

Join the tips of your Index finger and Thumb together and press slightly.

Keep all the other fingers extended outwards as shown in the image.

After forming the Mudras on both the hands, hold the Mudra made by your right hand in front of your heart and rest the Mudra made your left hand on your left knee.

Relax your shoulders.

Duration:

This Mudra should be performed for at least 5 minutes and can be performed for 40 minutes at a stretch.

This Mudra should be performed twice a day, once in the morning and once in the evening for best results.

Mudra #9

Sahastraarmudra / Mudra of Thousand Petals

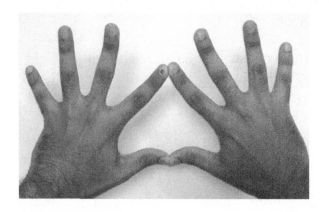

Method:

This Mudra can be performed while being seated or in a standing position.

Concentrate on your breathing to relax and feel comfortable.

Raise your hands at chest height, with your palms facing down.

Now, join the tips of both the Index fingers together and press slightly.

Then, join the tips of both the Thumbs together forming a Triangle. (Refer the image)

Keep all the other fingers extended and outstretched.

Once you have formed this Mudra, raise the Mudra at a height of around 6 inches above your head.

And now visualize as if a shower of light and energy are entering the top of your head through the triangle formed in the Mudra.

Duration:

This Mudra should be performed for at least 5 minutes and can be performed for 20 minutes at a stretch.

This Mudra should be performed twice a day, once in the morning and once in the evening for best results.

Mudra #10

Vyaanamudra / Mudra of Omnipresent Integration

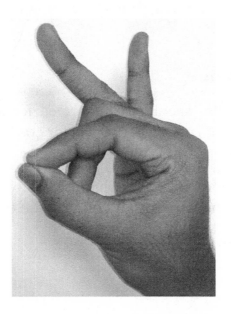

Method:

This Mudra is to be performed in a seated position.

Be seated comfortably in an upright posture and concentrate on your breathing to relax.

Advait

Join the tips of the Thumb and the Index finger and press slightly.

Touch the tip of the Middle finger to the midline of the Thumb. (Refer the image)

Keep the Ring and Little fingers extended upwards.

Once the Mudra is formed on both the hands, place it in your lap, palms facing upwards.

Duration:

This Mudra should be performed for at least 5 minutes and can be performed for 40 minutes at a stretch.

This Mudra should be performed twice a day, once in the morning and once in the evening for best results.

Mudra #11

Kashyapmudra / Mudra of Turtle

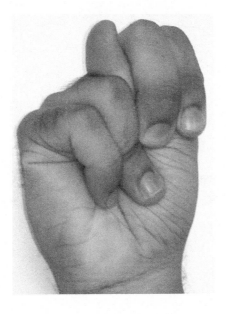

Method:

This Mudra is to be performed in a seated position.

Be seated comfortably in an upright posture and concentrate on your breathing to relax.

Advait

Drive the tip of your Thumb through the space between the Middle and the Ring finger.

Now, fold down all the other fingers to make a fist, with the tip of your Thumb sticking out.

After forming this Mudra on both your hands, place them on your thighs and relax your chest and belly.

Duration:

This Mudra should be performed for at least 5 minutes and can be performed for 40 minutes at a stretch.

This Mudra should be performed twice a day, once in the morning and once in the evening for best results.

Mudra #12

Mustikamudra / Mudra of Joined Fists

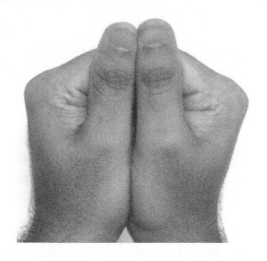

Method:

This Mudra is to be performed in a seated position.

Be seated comfortably in an upright posture and concentrate on your breathing to relax.

Raise your palms to chest height facing you.

Advait

Now, try to touch the heel of your palms (base of the palm) with the tips of all the fingers with your Thumbs extended upwards.

Now make the palms face each other and then join them together with the thumbs touching each other sideways. (Refer the image)

After forming the Mudra, hold it against your chest.

Relax your shoulders, neck and throat.

Duration:

This Mudra should be performed for at least 5 minutes and can be performed for 25 minutes at a stretch.

This Mudra should be performed twice a day, once in the morning and once in the evening for best results.

Mudra #13

Hridaymudra / Mudra of Heart

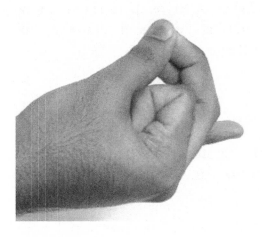

Method:

This Mudra is to be performed in a seated position.

Be seated comfortably in an upright posture and concentrate on your breathing to relax.

Try to touch the base of the Index finger with the tip of the same Index finger.

Advait

Now, roll this bent Index finger forward in such a way that the first knuckle of the Index finger touches the base of the Thumb (Refer the image).

Now join the tips of the Thumb, Middle and Ring fingers together and press slightly.

Keep the Little finger outstretched.

This Mudra is to be performed on both your palms simultaneously and then rest this Mudras on your thighs.

Duration:

This Mudra should be performed for at least 5 minutes and can be performed for 40 minutes at a stretch.

This Mudra should be performed twice a day, once in the morning and once in the evening for best results.

Mudra #14

Pralambmudra / Mudra of Garland

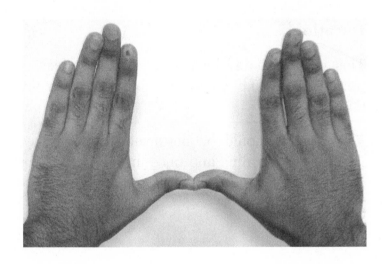

Method:

This Mudra is to be performed in a seated position.

Be seated comfortably in an upright posture and concentrate on your breathing to relax.

Raise your palms to chest height with the palms facing down.

Advait

Now, touch the tips of both the Thumbs together and press slightly.

Keep all the other fingers extended and touching each other adjacently.

(Refer the image for more clarity)

Duration:

This Mudra should be performed for at least 5 minutes and can be performed for 30 minutes at a stretch.

This Mudra should be performed twice a day, once in the morning and once in the evening for best results.

Mudra #15

Pratham Uttarbodhimudra / Mudra of Supreme Awakening I

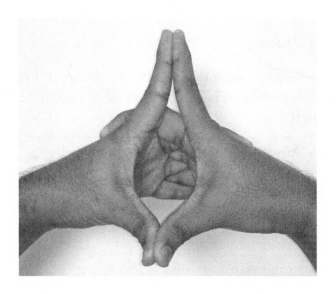

Method:

This Mudra can be performed while being seated, in a standing position or lying in bed.

Concentrate on your breathing to relax and feel comfortable.

Interlace the fingers of both the hands together.

Now join the tips of the Index finger and the Thumbs together as shown in the image and extend the Index fingers as upwards as possible, simultaneously extending the Thumbs downwards.

(Refer the image for clarity.)

Duration:

This Mudra should be performed for at least 5 minutes and can be performed for 40 minutes at a stretch.

This Mudra should be performed twice a day, once in the morning and once in the evening for best results.

Mudra #16

Dwitiiya Uttarbodhimudra / Mudra of Supreme Awakening II

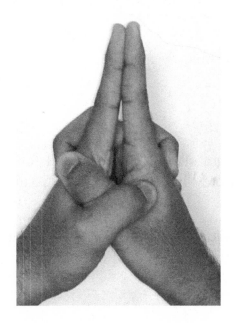

Method:

This Mudra is to be performed in a sitting position.

Be seated comfortably in an upright posture and concentrate on your breathing to relax.

Clasp your hands together, and interlace the fingers of both the hands together.

Now join the tips of the Index finger as shown in the image and extend the Index fingers as upwards as possible,

Then cross-over the left Thumb on the right Thumb.

(Refer the image)

Duration:

This Mudra should be performed for at least 5 minutes and can be performed for 40 minutes at a stretch.

This Mudra should be performed twice a day, once in the morning and once in the evening for best results.

*Note:

This Mudra was used by ancient Indian Maharshi's / Yogi's for attracting inspiration and insight.

This Mudra strengthens the willpower and increases your focus towards achieving your aim.

Mudra #17

Garudamudra / Mudra of Eagle

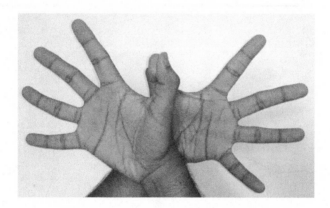

Method:

This Mudra can be performed while being seated, in a standing position or lying in bed.

Concentrate on your breathing to relax and feel comfortable.

Bring both your hands in front of your chest, palms facing the chest.

Cross the hands with the right hand crossing over the left hand and interlock the Thumbs at the first padding. (Refer the image)

Mudras for Anxiety

Keep all the other fingers extended and outstretched.

Create a firm pressure between the pads of the Thumb.

Duration:

This Mudra should be performed for at least 5 minutes and can be performed for 40 minutes at a stretch.

This Mudra should be performed twice a day, once in the morning and once in the evening for best results.

Mudra #18

Hamsimudra / Mudra of Spirit Contained

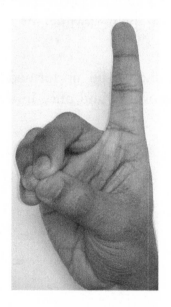

Method:

This Mudra can be performed while being seated, in a standing position or lying in bed.

Concentrate on your breathing to relax and feel comfortable.

Mudras for Anxiety

Join the tips of your Middle finger, Ring finger, Little finger and Thumb together and press slightly.

Keep the Index finger extended outwards.

Duration:

No specific duration, perform as long as you wish, or, as long as it takes to achieve the desired effect.

Best results are obtained when performed for 15 minutes at a stretch.

Mudra #19

AbhayHridaymudra / Mudra of Assured Heart

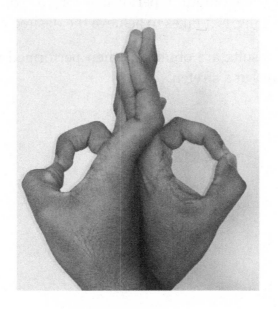

Method:

This Mudra is to be performed in a seated position.

Be seated comfortably in an upright posture and concentrate on your breathing to relax.

Mudras for Anxiety

Join your palms together as in the Indian form of salutation 'Namaste'.

Now cross the palms at your wrist, with the back of the palms facing each other and the wrist of the right hand closer to the body.

Interlock the Index, Middle and Little fingers at the tips. (Refer the image)

Join the tips of the Ring fingers and the Thumbs as shown in the image.

Duration:

This Mudra should be performed for at least 5 minutes and can be performed for 45 minutes at a stretch.

This Mudra should be performed twice a day, once in the morning and once in the evening for best results.

Advait

Mudra #20

Padmamudra / Mudra of Lotus

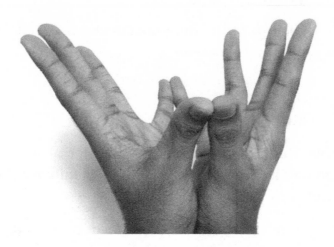

Method:

This Mudra is to be performed in a seated position.

Be seated comfortably in an upright posture and concentrate on your breathing to relax.

Touch the Thumb and Little finger of the left hand to the Thumb and Little finger of the right hand.

Join the base of both the palms together.

Mudras for Anxiety

Stretch all the other fingers outwards and keep them straight.

Refer the image above.

This Mudra should be held in front of your chest.

Duration:

This Mudra should be performed for at least 5 minutes and can be performed for 40 minutes at a stretch.

This Mudra should be performed twice a day, once in the morning and once in the evening for best results.

Mudra #21

Mudgaramudra / Mudra of the Club

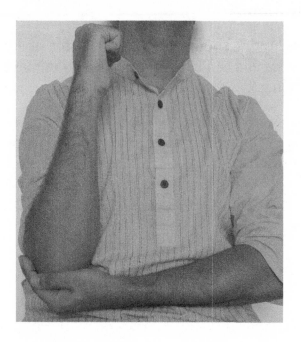

Method:

This Mudra is to be performed in a seated position.

Be seated comfortably in an upright posture and concentrate on your breathing to relax.

Mudras for Anxiety

Form a fist with your right hand and rest the right elbow on the left palm.

(Refer the image)

Relax the shoulders and breathe comfortably.

Duration:

This Mudra should be performed for at least 5 minutes and can be performed for 30 minutes at a stretch.

This Mudra should be performed twice a day, once in the morning and once in the evening for best results.

Advait

Mudra #22

Kilakmudra / Mudra of Bondage

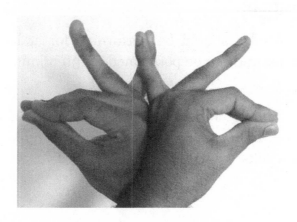

Method:

This Mudra is to be performed in a seated position.

Be seated comfortably in an upright posture and concentrate on your breathing to relax.

Cross your wrists with the back of your palms facing each other.

Mudras for Anxiety

Now stretch out both the Little fingers, and then hook them with their tips touching and pressing against each other. (Refer the image)

Lift up both the ring fingers, slightly.

Join the tips of the Thumb, Index and Middle fingers on both the hands together.

Duration:

This Mudra should be performed for at least 5 minutes and can be performed for 45 minutes at a stretch.

This Mudra should be performed twice a day, once in the morning and once in the evening for best results.

Mudra #23

Ganeshmudra / Mudra of Lord Ganesh (The Elephant God)

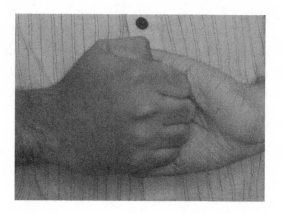

Method:

This Mudra can be performed while being seated, in a standing position or lying in bed.

Concentrate on your breathing to relax and feel comfortable.

Bring your palms in front of your chest. Your left palm must be facing outward while the right palm must be facing your chest.

Mudras for Anxiety

Form a 'hook' by bending your fingers.

Now hook the hands together by clasping as shown in the image.

Pull gently to exert slight pressure on the fingers.

Hold the Mudra in front of your chest.

Duration:

This Mudra should be performed for at least 5 minutes and can be performed for 20 minutes at a stretch.

This Mudra should be performed twice a day, once in the morning and once in the evening for best results.

Mudra #24

Tritiiya Varahamudra / Mudra of Hog III

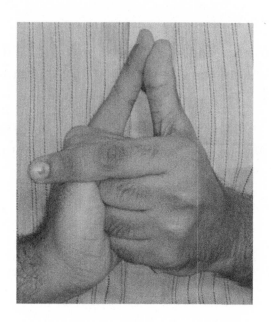

Method:

This Mudra is to be performed in a seated position.

Be seated comfortably in an upright posture and concentrate on your breathing to relax.

Mudras for Anxiety

Hold your left hand in front of your chest, palm facing you.

Curl the Middle, Ring and Little finger of the left hand inwards.

The Index finger should be pointing towards right and the Thumb should be extended upwards.

Now, clasp the curled fingers of the left hand with the fingers of the right hand.

Then, touch the tip of the Thumb of your left hand with the tip of the Index finger of your right hand.

Touch the tip of your right Thumb to the base of the left Thumb.

The Left Index finger should be resting outside the right Little finger.

Duration:

This Mudra should be performed for at least 5 minutes and can be performed for 45 minutes at a stretch.

This Mudra should be performed twice a day, once in the morning and once in the evening for best results.

Mudra #25

Chakramudra / Mudra of Wheel

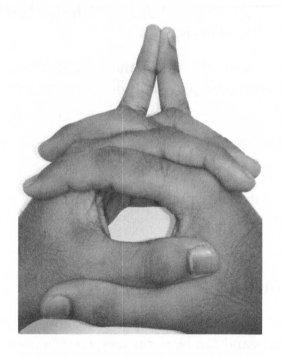

Method:

This Mudra is to be performed in a seated position.

Mudras for Anxiety

Be seated comfortably in an upright posture and concentrate on your breathing to relax.

Interlace your fingers together as shown in the image.

Extend both your Ring fingers upwards, then touch the tips of these two fingers and press slightly.

This Mudra is to be held in front of your navel.

Duration:

This Mudra should be performed for at least 5 minutes and can be performed for 40 minutes at a stretch.

This Mudra should be performed twice a day, once in the morning and once in the evening for best results.

Thank You

Thank you so much for reading my book. I hope you really liked it.

As you probably know, many people look at the reviews on Amazon before they decide to purchase a book.

If you liked the book, please take a minute to leave a review with your feedback.

60 seconds is all I'm asking for, and it would mean a lot to me.

Thank You so much.

All the best,

Advait

Other Books by Advait

Mudras for Awakening Chakras: 19 Simple Hand Gestures for Awakening & Balancing Your Chakras

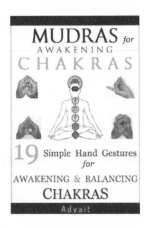

http://www.amazon.com/dp/B00P82COAY

[#1 Bestseller in 'Yoga']

[#1 Bestseller in 'Chakras']

Mudras for Weight Loss: 21 Simple Hand
Gestures for Effortless Weight Loss

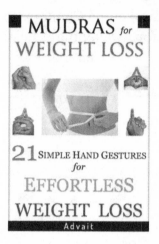

http://www.amazon.com/dp/B00P3ZPSEK

Mudras for Spiritual Healing: 21 Simple Hand Gestures for Ultimate Spiritual Healing & Awakening

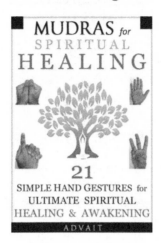

http://www.amazon.com/dp/B00PFYZLQO

Mudras for Sex: 25 Simple Hand Gestures for
Extreme Erotic Pleasure & Sexual Vitality

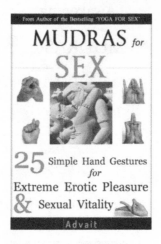

Mudras for Anxiety

Mudras: 25 Ultimate Techniques for Self Healing

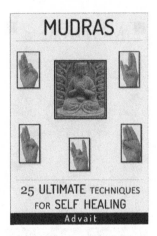

http://www.amazon.com/dp/B00MMPB5CI

Mudras for a Strong Heart: 21 Simple Hand
Gestures for Preventing, Curing & Reversing
Heart Disease

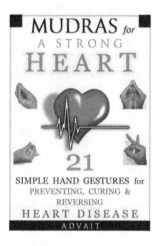

http://www.amazon.com/dp/B00PFRLGTM

Mudras for Anxiety

Mudras for Curing Cancer: 21 Simple Hand Gestures for Preventing & Curing Cancer

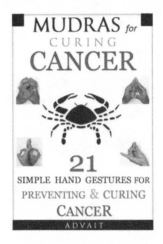

http://www.amazon.com/dp/B00PFO199M

Mudras for Stress Management: 21 Simple Hand
Gestures for a Stress Free Life

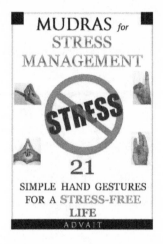

http://amazon.com/dp/B00PFTJ6OC

Mudras for Anxiety

Mudras for Memory Improvement: 25 Simple Hand Gestures for Ultimate Memory Improvement

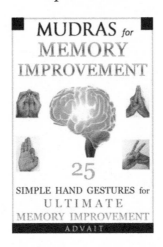

http://www.amazon.com/dp/B00PFSP8TK

Made in United States
North Haven, CT
10 August 2023

40171705R00050